# How to Adapt Paleo
# To Your Life

Jitka Egressy

ISBN: 1508487197
ISBN-13: 978-1508487197

To everyone who wants to life better.

# CONTENTS

# ABOUT THE AUTHOR

Jitka Egressy is a passionate cook and wife. She loves creating variations of meals that are both healthy and tasty. She is the kind of a person who loves enjoying every single bite.

Jitka has a comprehensive knowledge of contemporary food allergies and specializes in creating easy, healthy and delicious recipes that are gluten-free, dairy-free and Paleo-friendly. She has more than 10 years of experience with many different diets and nutrition plans.

Those days are gone when her most devoted audience was her husband, colleagues and friends. Jitka is sharing her ideas and recipes with her favorite readers on her blog, the name of which can't be anything other than: http://www.easyhealthyandyummy.com/

**Other eBooks from Jitka Egressy:**

Paleo Cookbook for Life: http://amzn.to/15FrKBr
Paleo Breakfast Ideas: http://amzn.to/1z3LfR7
Rainbow Smoothies: http://amzn.to/1GNTK6d
10 EASY STEPS TO START HEALTHY LIFESTYLE RIGHT NOW:
http://amzn.to/1xPOE1K

# 1 WHAT IS PALEO

The name Paleo originates from the Paleolithic era. It refers to a modern nutritional diet designed to emulate, insofar as possible using modern foods, the diet of wild plants and animals eaten by humans during this era.

It's mainly based on avoiding the consumption of dairy, grains, legumes, processed oils and refined sugar.

Here is link for you, if you want more information about Perfect Health Diet check out amazing book from Paul Jaminet: http://amzn.to/1B351fO

## What to Eat and What to Avoid

### The Okay List (food that you should eat on a daily basis)

Meat - choose grass-fed and pastured meats.
Chicken, turkey, beef, pork, lamb - even venison!
Eggs - again, go for organic every time is possible
Wild-caught seafood
Vegetables
Avocado oil, olive oil, coconut oil - in the best quality possible.

**The Moderation List**

Fruits
Nuts (peanuts are not nuts, it's legume so avoid those)
Nut oils
Seeds

Safe starches - white rice, white potatoes or sweet potatoes (about 400 cal per day maximum; note that, according to the Perfect Health Diet, which is what I follow, starches are not Paleo)

**The Avoid It List**

All grains, including corn and soybeans
Legumes
Dairy
Sugar
Processed foods
Vegetable oils

# 2 HOW TO START WITH PALEO

## 1. Think different

The most difficult thing about starting Paleo is changing your mind. We have heard for decades that low fat is okay for us. It can be hard to start thinking different... I love that commercial from Apple "Think different" so I borrowed this slogan. :-)

So forget about low fat labels! Don't be afraid of fats anymore! The key is choosing good fat and avoiding bad fat. Enjoy bacon again! Just grab your veggies too, please. Don't use margarine - it's chemicals, not real food. Prepare ghee instead (check my cookbook for the recipe if you want). Use olive oil, coconut oil, flaxseed oil (in moderation) or ghee. Even fat from the bacon you prepared for breakfast can be used. Save it for later. :-)

On the other hand avoid vegetable oils such sunflower oil, soybean oil, canola oil...

Try new meats you've never eaten before. Liver, beef belly, beef tail, ... The principle "eat animal nose to tail" is going strong here. Use bones from lunch to prepare nourishing bone broth. Eat marrow - it's delicious and full of nutrients.

Eat more veggies! Choose fresh greens for your meals. You can eat as many veggies as you want. It's a big part of my plate with every meal I eat. Fill about half of your plate with fresh, organic veggies if possible. Add a good source of protein like chicken, beef, lamb or fish then add a smaller portion of good fat like avocado or a few nuts, smaller pieces of fruit and you are good to go.

Remove all processed foods first. This is huge step, I know. But definitely worth it!

Change your mind about traditional meals. Bread is only a "vehicle" for ham and veggies. Eat just the ham and veggies. What is the main component in Spaghetti Bolognese? Pasta or tomato sauce with meat? Of course it's the sauce with meat. Can you eat only pasta with nothing added? NO! It's not delicious at all. But can you eat Bolognese sauce with meat only? YES! How yummy!

Breakfast is not only granola with milk or toast with butter and jam! Think different and enjoy dinner for breakfast and breakfast for dinner. There is no rule limiting you to not eat chicken with veggies for breakfast or scrambled eggs with bacon for dinner!

Another new part of your life will be leftovers. Celebrate them! Leftovers can save you time. Plan them! When you cook any meal, prepare more portions than needed and save them for another day!

Cooking Paleo is easier than you think. I will show you later in this book.

## 2. Cleanse challenge

When you start on Paleo you should begin with a cleanse challenge. Why? You need to know your body. You need to know how your body reacts to different types of food. This is the best way to prepare your own meal plan according to your body. Each of us is a unique organism and we need unique diets too.

I can recommend this great book for your cleansing period.

Perfect Health Diet by Paul Jaminet: http://amzn.to/1B351fO
21-Day Paleo Cleanse: https://www.paleoplan.com/21-day-paleo-cleanse-ebook/

Intro to Paleo: Quick-Start Diet Guide to Burn Fat, Lose Weight, and Build Muscle from Abel James and George Bryant: http://amzn.to/1Dm26Ow

I highly recommend you do NOT skip the cleansing period. I know, it can be hard but it's worth it. Believe me. I started my Paleo journey with a cleansing period too and this was such an amazing opportunity to feel my body. I listened to my body and removed all food that doesn't work for me. My diet changed the person I am. I feel great now and this changed my attitude too.

This way you can create your own diet, which can be followed for the rest of your life. Paleo is a type of lifestyle. It's not about a short period when you are targeting your goal weight. Paleo is about health and natural eating which makes you happy and healthy. So please invest in yourself for this short cleansing period. It's your life, your health, your happiness.....

## 3. Clean your home

You need to clean your body, but you also need to clean our home. Remove all foods that are not Paleo friendly. If you will not eat them, why do you need them at home? Remove all processed food, junk food, flour, refined sugar, all frozen pizzas. You CAN cut them out.... you can.

Unopened foods which are still okay can be donated to your local charities, for example. Opened food and food that cannot be donated, put in the trash. NOW! Yes, you really do not need those cookies for visitors! You can prepare healthier snacks for them if you want. No, you don't need candies for kids. Prepare fresh fruits for them instead. There is no real reason to save food that makes you sick!

This is your new starting point. Enjoy every step. You can do everything better now. Be happy to clean your house. It's not a waste. It's saving your life, your health and happiness.

# 3 HOW TO SHOP PALEO

## 1. When to shop

You have to change your shopping habits and this is another huge step. I think that clean shopping is the most powerful piece in the whole process of your transformation.

Why? It's simple. You will not eat crap if you do not buy crap. Your house is already clear, right? Then you have at home only "clean" food.

If you do not buy any other crap, than you will cook and eat better food. Yes! It's that simple. But wait a minute... you have to be strong. It's not as easy as you think.

Maybe you are strong now, but what about when you hit your local supermarket? You might even be hungry, which makes you crazy and you will make bad decisions.

So my first bit of advice is:

### DO NOT GO SHOPPING WHEN YOU ARE HUNGRY!

Cliché? Truth! If you are hungry, your brain is working differently.

## 2. How to shop

Use a list. I am serious! Write a list for yourself - on paper, in your phone, I don't care - just prepare yourself for shopping. What do you need for cooking for next week? Make a list and stick with it. Do not buy anything else. This will help you for the beginning period.

If you create a "clean" shopping list and stick with it, than you cannot buy anything wrong, right? If you don't have on your list granola, why visit the section with colorful boxes (full of sugar and other crap). NO, those candies are not on your list either! Put them down!

I think you get idea. A shopping list can help you with "emotional shopping" - when you see candies, you want candies, etc.

If you don't have a shopping list, go to the "fresh" goods first.

Veggie and fruit corner - you should fill your basket mainly here. Plan vegetable and fruit for every meal = 2 - 3 portions a day.

Meat, poultry and eggs - grab enough protein for your meals.

Then grab some olive oil, coconut oil and maybe a few batches of nuts or seeds.

That's it! No need to go to the "candies corner" or corner with potato chips...

Why would you want to buy ice cream, if you don't plan to eat it??
- it's nonsense
- if you avoid it, you are further in a single step
- tell your family for help - do not buy crap for them either

**So again, in short:**
- do not go shopping when you are hungry
- make a shopping list and stick with it
- plan your week (buying meat once a week)
- plan which meals you will cook, then buy food only for those meals
- omit "bad corners" = do not even go there
- do not buy what you should avoid

Okay, maybe you really need to shop for different food for your family. But please split your fridge if necessary - 2 parts, yours and your family - and be strong. Do not even check the family part! It's not food for you. Use the same technique for the cupboard, too.

If you cook for your family and they are not Paleo eaters, cook a Paleo version, remove your portion (and maybe anything as a leftover for next days) and then add the "dirty" ingredients.

So you get your clean food + leftovers and your family gets the comfort food they enjoy.

## 3. Choose organic

If you can, choose organic vegetables, fruits, meat, poultry and eggs when possible. Organic food is always better for you. No, or lower, pesticides, no hormones in the meat, eggs from grass fed chicken.

Give it a chance. Try organic and you will never go back. Organic tastes better - believe me. Plus you will get better (read healthier) food for your body.

It's worth spending a few bucks more here.

If you need to save some money go with organic for these:

1. Apples
2. Strawberries
3. Grapes
4. Celery
5. Peaches
6. Spinach
7. Sweet Bell Peppers
8. Nectarines (Imported)
9. Cucumbers
10. Cherry Tomatoes
11. Potatoes
12. Hot Peppers
13. Kale/Collard Greens

These produce picks contain the lowest pesticide levels:

1. Avocados
2. Pineapples
3. Cabbage
4. Onions
5. Asparagus
6. Mangoes
7. Papayas
8. Kiwi
9. Eggplant
10. Grapefruit
11. Cantaloupe
12. Cauliflower
13. Sweet Potatoes

So it's okay to buy those in not organic quality.

## 4. Read labels

It's really important to read labels! Producers are trying to fool us with BIG colorful labels in the front... but turn the package over. Read the ingredients list and you will quickly put it back on the shelf when you notice chemicals, sugar and such a long list of non-readable ingredients in your favorite snack, believe me.

You need to check everything - sure, the best foods are those without a list of ingredients - vegetables, fruit, meat, poultry, eggs...

Be sure to check your juice! Is it really 100% juice with no added sugar? Not made from concentrate?

Check your favorite mayonnaise! It's full of crap, right? Make it yourself if you like it.

The fewer ingredients in the list, the better! If anything has more than, let's say, 6-7 ingredients, don't buy it. It's usually full of chemicals.

If you cannot read or pronounce any of the ingredients, don't buy it. What is Ferrous sulfate? Do you know it? No? Then don't buy it.

# 4 HOW TO COOK PALEO

## 1. Change your habits

You have to change your mind. You will cook a completely different way. Start planning your meals. You have to plan your leftovers.

Seems to be a lot of work? Don't worry; I have a great plan for you. You need to spend only 2 hours a week in your kitchen to eat amazing food for the whole work week. Yes, it's possible. Forgot about fancy 4 hours whatever books :-) This is real. I have been following this plan for about a year now with no problems. Let me change your mind... Cooking is not time consuming, if you plan everything ahead of time.

This is how it works for me:

I have two cooking session. The first is Sunday evening (one hour) and then Wednesday evening (one hour). That's it. Sure, I cook more often during weekends - but only if I want something special for my hubby.

**First session** (for me it's Sunday, but choose any day that works for you)

I cook a few portions of rice and potatoes (since I'm a Perfect health diet eater - moderation of safe starches). Split portions into food containers and put them in the fridge. During the week I can easily pair them with protein and vegetable to get my meal done in a minute.

I also prepare some "ready to eat" meals. Usually 4 portions (2 for me and 2 for my hubby). So I bake chicken legs, or beef and split them into food containers with my rice or potatoes, add some fresh veggies and put them into the fridge again.

Then I bake some veggies like carrots with chili peppers, zucchini, onions even mushrooms as a side for my meals.

So by the end of this one-hour session I typically have:
- 4-6 portions of my safe starches
- 4-6 portions of fresh or steamed veggie and mushrooms
- 4-6 portions of protein - chicken, beef, lamb, livers, hard boiled eggs

I usually prepare 4 ready to eat meals = one portion of safe starches, one portion of protein and one portion of veggies into a single food container.

The rest of my starches, veggies and proteins I leave separated so I can combine them according to my actual taste.

**Second session** (for me it's Wednesday, but again choose any day that works for you)

Ok, during my second session I usually prepare only a few portions ahead. Like 2-3 portions, since I usually cook fresh food during the weekends, or I'm not home during the weekend at all.

So by the end of this one-hour session I typically have:
- 2-3 portions of my safe starches
- 2-3 portions of fresh or steamed veggie and mushrooms
- 2-3 portions of protein - chicken, beef, lamb, livers, hard boiled eggs

I try to make a fresh combination every time. So if I go for chicken and beef on Monday, then I prepare lamb and livers with hard boiled eggs on Wednesday. Same with veggies.

If I have more time I prepare something like egg muffins or even pizza. But I usually stick with "easy to reheat" meals. I grab them in the morning to take with me to work and reheat them in a microwave when it's time for lunch.

For my breakfast I usually go for smoothies during the week, since it's super easy and fast for preparation, and gives me so much energy in the morning. I have a booklet about smoothies, so check it out on Amazon, if you want: Rainbow Smoothies http://amzn.to/1GNTK6d

During the weekends I love big breakfasts. Almost brunches. Like eggs with bacon and lots of veggies. I love a long lazy breakfast on weekends, but during the work week I need to be ready pretty fast in the morning.

## 2. Love leftovers

Leftovers are amazing. If you plan them, you can save a lot of your time! For example are you baking a chicken for your family? Put two of them in the oven at the same time. You will get an amazing dinner for your family and also lunches for the next 1-2 days.

Save with sides. Make everything in bigger batches in order to get leftovers. Then you can combine them with other leftovers or make only a part of your meal fresh. If you save sides from dinner for another day, then you can freshly prepare "only" meat.

Same for chili con carne (I make them without beans and with lot of fresh tomatoes), or Bolognese sauce for my zucchini noodles. I cook about 8 portions in my slow cooker, pack 4 of them into food containers for the next few days and freeze the other 4 for the next week or so. If I have no time, my freezer is full of great homemade food to grab and enjoy!

I think you get the idea.

## 3. Lunches to go

I always plan my lunches ahead. I hate eating out on a daily basis. I don't like making compromises in "classic" restaurants. And usually don't have time to in the office. So it's 2 in 1, baby. :)

I get amazing food, have 100% control over it and save a lot of time! I can eat healthy and balanced meals every day.

Sometimes you don't have the opportunity to reheat your meal, right? So you have to figure out lunches to go, which can be eaten (and stored) everywhere. A typical example is flights. I hate food plane food. It's not good for your health and tastes awful. It's also full of chemical; no thanks. I can have something like hardboiled egg with carrots, almonds, baked chicken, lettuce wraps, egg muffins...

Get it? It's not so hard. Just make a plan and you are fine.

## 4. Slow cooker - your best friend

I mentioned before that I use my slow cooker. Actually - I love it! It's such an amazing tool! You can put ingredients inside, turn it on, go to work and when you come back and it's time for dinner, your slow cooker prepared amazing food. It's done when you hit the door!

Isn't this amazing? Fresh, warm meals with no work.

Bone broth is amazing from a slow cooker too. Again no work, no checking, you can go to work and the slow cooker is working for you...

I have a full blog post about slow cookers so check it out here: http://www.easyhealthyandyummy.com/2014/11/slow-cooker-is-it-worthy.html

## 5. Baking

Oh yes, you can still enjoy baked goods on Paleo. It's not the same, but don't worry it can be done.

We have so many flour substitutes these days. You can use:
- almond flour
- coconut flour
- tapioca flour
- macadamia flour
- chestnut flour
- etc.

Check out your local store. Many of these you can even prepare at home - like almond flour.

You can find amazing recipes on the Internet or even in my eBooks (Paleo Cookbook for Life - http://amzn.to/15FrKBr).

Yes, it will take time to experiment with different preparations, but it's worth it. Don't forget that it's still a treat! Sweets should not be part of your daily meals.

# 5 HOW TO DEAL WITH EATING OUT

So far you prepare your food at home, eat clean and feel amazing. What if your friends invite you to a restaurant for dinner? Don't worry, it's okay! You can live a "normal" social life and still eat healthy!

When you are eating out, you can still try to eat as healthy as possible.

It's about preparation - prepare yourself ahead of time! If it's possible, check the menu of the restaurant in advance on their website. Many restaurants have their menus online, so choose your meal before even getting to the restaurant. Choose a steak and veggie salad or fish with steamed vegetables. Prepare yourself to make preparation requests of the waiter. Do you want to remove dressing from your salad? Ask for it! Do you want to replace French fries with sautéed veggies? Do it! Ask for your healthier options.

If the waiter tells you it's not possible to make any changes then you have two options - leave (not the best choice when it's dinner with friends) or order the healthiest possible option and eat only the meat and veggies. Remove the croutons from your salad; don't eat French fries ... Remember, it's about choices. You can resist!

I still believe that eating out is a great opportunity to be social, so don't give up. It takes time to be strong enough to resist and find your way to eat as healthy as possible.

My favorite types of restaurants are:

## 1. American
- no bun hamburgers with sweet potato fries - super easy to order, you can add a veggie side and you are fine
- steak with vegetables - amazing decision here

## 2. Mexican
- Burrito Bowl/Naked Burrito, hold the beans and tortillas or rice, order extra guacamole

## 3. Italian
- sure, there is pasta and pizza, but also great salads with chicken or shrimp
- you can find steaks here too
- fresh starters

## 4. Thai
- you can find soups or curry sauce made from coconut milk with grilled veggies

In summary: take out the bad carbs and replace them with good ones.

# 6 HOW TO TELL YOUR FRIENDS ABOUT PALEO

All of us know those situations well - you start a new lifestyle and your friends recognize changes and start to ask you...

You tell them about Paleo and here is where the problems start. They start calling you caveman or even worse. Ask you if you hunt for your steaks, etc.

You need a lot of patience!

**Do not judge them**

You didn't know about Paleo a few months ago either. Do you remember how you skeptical you were at first? They are too!

Everyone needs time to change their mind. It's not an easy thing at all. If they are curious about your lifestyle it's actually a good thing! Lack of interest means they don't care about you. So be happy that they care about your new lifestyle.

You can give them all the information about Paleo. You can tell them how it works for you, for your body. You can even tell them about the fun parts (jokes about caveman, etc.). But never ever tell them that they are doing it wrong and the only correct way is yours.

## Be patient

It can take time until your friends will see results on you. Your body, your mind, your energy level... then they will start changing their minds - maybe. They will start to ask you how you eat Paleo.

Their questions will become more specific - how you stay on Paleo during work lunches, for example.

This is a great point. They start to thinking about Paleo and how they can adapt it. This is your chance to guide them, help them. Be their guide! Tell them about your journey to a Paleo lifestyle. Share with them this book, for example.

Tell them your own hacks. Show them your favorite restaurants; give them tips on how to stay in budget on Paleo... anything!

## Answer questions

Answer every question patiently. You know everything you need. They have just the information from newspapers or TV. Maybe even only from "one guy told me".

Some people need to know the science part of this lifestyle. Recommend books, websites, forums... Show them your life!

Be patient with "stupid" questions. They seem to be stupid for you, but maybe not for them. Maybe they are asking something they are genuinely concerned about.

## Be guide

If they decide to try it, be their guide. Share your lunch with them. Invite them to your favorite restaurant and show them how you order your meal to stay Paleo.

Go shopping together. You can give them useful information about how to shop, how to save some money, where they can shop, etc.

This is your chance to change their life. They can be healthier if you have enough patience. It's worth it, isn't it?

**Never give up**

There will be situations when you would like to scream or run away. For sure. I had many of them. People don't believe in Paleo until they try it on their own. I had very painful situations with the father of my hubby. He is a traditional eater, believes in traditional eating pyramids with grains as the biggest part, in doctors who say we should eat whole grains five times a day, etc.

But I never gave up. You know why? It's your life! It's your body! It's your health we are talking about! This effort is definitely worth it if you feel better, look better, live better..., isn't it?

You have to be strong! This is not easy. I know.

I recommend starting with Paleo on your own. Do not tell your friends until you are ready. You have to believe in your lifestyle before they try to ruin your opinion.

# 7 RESOURCES

My favorite blogs about Paleo/PHD:

www.nomnompaleo.com– great site with tons of recipes, an app for your mobile phone, funny cartoon Michelle and much more

www.paleomg.com– lovely Juli, I really love her every post

www.ontherun.barborkas.cz– hard worker, runner, inspiration – that is Barborka

For more healthy recipes, ideas and a blog about my life, you can check my site: www.easyhealthyandyummy.com

Feel free send me any questions: easyhealthyandyummy@gmail.com

For my Instagram posts visit
www.instagram.com/easyhealthyandyummy

Follow me on Twitter: @JitkaEgressy

# 8 THANK YOU

I would like to thank you for purchasing my book.

I would love to get your feedback in the form of a review. Your honest reviews will continue to inspire me. Any review helps me a lot! Thank you for every word...

You can post a review on Amazon.com.

Check out my #1 Best Seller cookbooks in the Food Allergy category:
**Paleo cookbook for Life**: http://amzn.to/15FrKBr

Or small booklets from my **Paleo Recipes for Every Day series**:
http://www.amazon.com/gp/bookseries/B00SQOMJX8/
1. **Paleo Breakfast Ideas**: http://amzn.to/1z3LfR7
2. **Rainbow Smoothies**: http://amzn.to/1GNTK6d

Do you need little kick to start eating healthy? Check out my small booklet:
**10 EASY STEPS TO START HEALTHY LIFESTYLE RIGHT NOW**:
http://amzn.to/1xP0E1K

Enjoy your life....
Jitka Egressy

"Don't eat anything if it doesn't have a mother
or it didn't grow from the ground!"

www.ingramcontent.com/pod-product-compliance
Lightning Source LLC
Chambersburg PA
CBHW050528290526
45786CB00007B/2735